HOW TO LOSE 10 POUNDS OF WEIGHT IN 10 DAYS QUICKLY

LEARN TO BURN FAT WITHOUT DOING A LOT OF EXERCISE, LOSE POUNDS NATURALLY, FOREVER AND WITHOUT REBOUND

ELIMINATE ABDOMINAL AND BODY FAT QUICKLY FROM THE COMFORT OF YOUR HOME, WITHOUT GYM

Jessy M. Brown

Índice

Introduction

Losing weight can be one of the most difficult things a person has to do. Like smoking, food is sometimes an addition. There are many reasons why someone may be overweight. In most cases, it is due to lack of exercise and eating the wrong foods. People often overeat out of habit. They can choose food informally throughout the day or eat snacks they love. In some cases, a woman has just had a child and needs to lose the excess weight she gained after having the baby. This can be difficult because a new baby is often exhausting and distressing to the body. It can be difficult to lose weight after giving birth, especially if you have other children to care for.

My weight gain problems didn't start

until I was older. I was a skinny boy all my life and even into adulthood. Even after I had my kids, in my 20s, I managed to lose weight using just a diet and a little exercise. I seemed to be one of the lucky ones who didn't have to struggle with the weight, although I saw many of my friends and family members trying to remove the excess weight. It helped that I had my kids at an earlier age and had them separated by almost three years - this gave my body a chance to get back in shape every time.

I remember when I turned 30, I started to feel like I was getting fat and I was doing it. A friend told me that after age 30, weight was harder to lose, so I joined a gym. I got back in shape. In fact, a good diet and exercise made me thinner than I was in high school. Although many people felt that at 1.70 meters and 118 pounds, I was too thin.   As the years went by, little by little I began to regain weight. After I turned 40, I began to see that it was even harder to lose weight. I went to another gym, got on a scale and saw that I weighed 155 pounds. This was more than I weighed when I gave birth to my daughter.

It was harder to lose weight after 40, but I managed. Then I turned 45 and it got even harder. For two years, I wasn't overweight, but I wasn't happy with my appearance. I no longer wore shorts or jeans and I wore elastic skirts all the time to hide the excess weight.   I would take some weight off, but then, during the winter months, especially during the holiday season, I would come back up. After the last holiday season, I realized that I had reached 145, mainly because I ate foods that were delicious, but not good for me. A sedentary lifestyle that we often have during the winter months also played into this fact.

This summer, however, I was determined to lose the weight I had gained and put back on my shorts that had been neglected for two summers. This time, however, I decided to do some research on weight loss and see which plans worked best. Naturally, I wanted to take off as much weight as possible in the shortest possible time. I was able to lose 10 pounds in 10 days using some of the tips in this book. Through diet and exercise, I then removed the remaining 9 pounds that were a little more than my weight loss goal and now fit into my shorts.

Losing 10 pounds in 10 days is not as hard as you think. Whether you just want to start a diet or if you are looking for a way to get rid of some vanity weight, the methods in this book I discuss are safe and will work for you. I also explore some unsafe ways in which some people will tell you that you work with weight loss and why you shouldn't try them as well as your ideal weight for your height and age. Many people, especially women, tend to have a distorted view of their bodies and what they should weigh. That's why before you try to lose weight, not only should you have a goal in mind, but you should also make sure that this goal is a healthy one that makes you look and feel better, as well as healthier, without looking emaciated.

Once you learn how to lose weight in this book, you'll also know how to maintain it. In addition to teaching you how to lose 10 pounds in 10 days, this book also teaches you how to live a healthier lifestyle, without having to go to the gym, buy special foods or spend money. After losing 10 pounds, you'll feel much more empowered about your body and your health.   Even if you have more weight to lose, this is a good start for taking that weight off and keeping it off.

Many weight loss programs will tell you that you should only lose 2 pounds a week if you are on a diet. The reason they tell you this is very simple - they want you to keep going to the program so you can keep paying. If you continue to follow the examples in this book, not only will you be able to lose 10 pounds in 10 days, but you can also continue to lose weight at an accelerated rate.

What to do and what not to do with your nutrition

Diet is the most important aspect of weight loss. What you eat is seen all over your body. Those who tell you that you can take a magic pill and eat all the garbage you want and still lose weight are lying to you to sell pills, which are usually dangerous.

If you really want to lose weight, there are certain foods you can eat, and certain foods you shouldn't eat. This doesn't mean you don't have to eat anything but rabbit food, but it does mean you have to stop eating that Big Mac with fries.

This entire book could be made up of foods that you shouldn't eat when you're on a diet. There are many foods that are delicious, but they are not good for you because they are high in fat or sugar. I'm going to concentrate on the foods that you will probably eat to give you some things that you should and shouldn't do with your diet.

Foods to avoid

The following are foods you should avoid when you are trying to lose 10 pounds in 10 days, or any time you are watching your weight. In fact, these foods are good to avoid... period:

- Fast food
- Fried foods
- Products marked low in fat or diet
- Cookies
- Sweets

- Cakes and other sweets
- Frozen foods

Please note that this list does not include words such as "carbohydrates" or "trans fats. This is because dieting to lose weight is not a complicated plan. You don't have to eliminate all the foods you eat or just eat protein, although you should increase your protein intake. You just have to avoid foods that are diet saboteurs.

Fast food

Fast foods are usually fried, greasy, high in fat, high in sugar, processed with chemicals, or high in sodium. The first thing you want to avoid when looking for a way to lose weight is fast food. That means any one of them. Many of them disguise themselves as "healthy foods".

They're not. For fast food giants like McDonald's to be able to offer salads, they have to be able to buy the ingredients so that they can be stored and distributed throughout the country. These "diet salads" often contain more calories than some of the sandwiches, especially if you add the dressing, which is usually high in fat and sugar.

Take your lunch. Even if you take a peanut butter sandwich from home, you're still getting fewer calories than you would if you ate in fast food restaurants. Actually, peanut butter, although it is fat, is very good for you as it is a good source of protein. You just don't want to exaggerate.

One of the first things you need to do if you are going to lose 10 pounds in 10 days is to give up the idea of eating out. Avoid the morning roll and lunch you eat at a fast-food restaurant in the afternoon. Take your lunch for 10 days and you will see a difference in your weight.

When I wanted to lose weight in the past, the first thing I did was remove McDonald's from my diet. I used to like McDonald's, but I knew that a Big Mac, an order of fries and a Coke had more calorie content than my body needed for a meal (that typical menu has 1300 calories). I never really liked counting calories and I prefer to do simple things, but I knew that the calories I consumed in fast food were more than the calories I consumed in the food I brought from home and they didn't really fill me up. Make eating fast food the first thing you eliminate if you're trying to lose weight.

Don't be fooled by Subway ads that say you can lose weight by eating your food. They consist of processed meats and cheeses that aren't good for you either. For fast food to be mass-produced as it is, it has to be treated with chemicals. If you want a vegetable sandwich, make it at home and bring it to work.

Fried food

Fried foods are delicious. Even the bugs would taste good if they were fried. But fried foods are high in fat, usually unsaturated. While many restaurants are getting rid of trans fats in their foods, due to demands from the FDA and other legal authorities, fried foods are high in fat and are not good for any diet. They're also high in calories. Eat grilled or barbecued foods if you want to lose weight and stay away from anything fried.

Many people eat fried foods because they are cheap and fill. But fried foods are one of the main reasons people get fat in the first place. They don't offer you the nutritional value you need for your body and the little value they have is diminished by the fact that they are fried. When cooking, use a George Foreman grill to make meats and even grilled vegetables. If you have to use some oil so that the food does not stick, use Extra Virgin Olive Oil.

Products marked low in fat or diet

Many people think they can eat so-called "diet" foods when they are on a diet. Stores are full of these foods that are usually loaded with chemicals and are often no better for you than regular foods. For example, Cheezits - one of my favorite snacks of all time. There is a variety of low fat Cheezits that I actually prefer to normal Cheezits. However, if you look at the fat and calorie content, you'll see that there's not much difference.

Snackwells are the same. These are cookies and low-fat cakes. What people don't realize is that they usually end up eating more of these foods because they feel they are "dietetic" foods. Foods that are sweet and marked as a dietetic food contain a sugar substitute (one of the many newer ones) that is worse for you than real sugar.

People tend to indulge excessively in the low-fat or diet snacks and foods out there, thinking they're getting away with it. While you can replace your regular foods with low-fat foods, you need to be aware of the chemicals that foods may contain, as well as the fact that they are not much lower in calories. If you have a Cheezits craving, have only a small portion of the low-fat type, but don't feel that because they are low-fat, you can eat the whole box.

You are better off having real foods at home than those that are marked as low in fat or diet, as you will not be tempted to overeat that sabotages your diet.

Biscuits, sweets, cakes and other sweets

Stay away from sugar if you want to lose 10 pounds in 10 days. Sugar is one of the main reasons people gain weight. Many people are greedy and can't stop eating these foods. Sugar is processed through the system very quickly. It is hard on the digestive organs and makes them work very hard to process food for elimination. Sugar stays in the bloodstream and becomes fat. While it can be difficult for anyone who likes sweet to stop eating it, it is essential that you do so if you want to lose weight.

   Sweets offer no nutritional value. They do nothing to help your body and are considered empty calories. You're eating them for nothing and they show up as fat in your body. Some diets tell you to avoid all foods that contain simple carbohydrates, such as bread. But while breads have nutritional value and at least fill, sweets offer nothing.   Nothing but calories that will accumulate in your body.

Frozen Foods

Lean Kitchen? Don't bother. Stay away from all frozen foods. They're loaded with sodium. They have to be loaded with sodium in order to keep them. Sodium will also make it retain water and make it harder for you to lose weight.   If you think the dietary foods you see in the frozen food aisle are your answer when it comes to losing weight, think again.   Not only do they have excessively small portions, but the sodium content negates the low calories of these foods.

By cooking at home and eating real foods, you can end up not only losing the weight you want to lose, but also eating healthier. Avoid fast foods, fried foods, sweets, dietetic foods and frozen foods if you want to lose weight.

Food to eat

When looking for foods to eat in your diet, look for natural foods. Also be careful when cooking them. You should also increase your protein intake so that your body burns more calories.

One important meal you don't want to miss is breakfast. You should eat protein for breakfast when you want to lose weight quickly as this will increase your metabolism and cause you to start burning fat early in the day. Breakfast foods should be high in protein, but should not contain sugar. Stay away from so-called protein bars.

Hard boiled eggs, grilled meats and whole grains are a good choice for breakfast. A boiled or poached egg is also a good choice when it comes to early foods because eggs are a good source of protein. Eggs have a bad reputation for being high in cholesterol, although this is not true. Egg whites are a good source of protein and as long as they are not fried, they are a good choice for breakfast.

Salads are good for lunch. You can try a low-fat dressing, although you can easily make your own salad dressing. Use Extra Virgin Olive Oil and Balsamic Vinegar and add herbs such as Oregano and Basil to the dressing and it will be low in fat and will not contain preservatives.   Grilled vegetables are also a good choice for lunch.

You want to add protein to your diet, but not too much fat.   The chicken breast is a good source of protein and if you handle it, you will get the benefits of protein without the fat. Fish is also an excellent source of protein, as is red meat. A burger without bread, for example, that has been grilled, will give you the protein you need for the day.

If you like candy, eat fruit. Although fruits have sugar, unlike sweets, they provide your body with the nutrients you need. Vegetables are also essential for a healthy diet. You can eat vegetables like celery and carrots all day - they have a minimum of calories and you actually spend more calories chewing on these vegetables than they contain.

In most cases, the foods you should eat when trying to lose weight are common sense. If you know what foods to stay away from, you should know what foods to eat. Cooking food is very important. You should cook at home instead of eating out and be careful with the oils and condiments you use. Simple substitutions, such as homemade burgers or chicken breasts for lunch instead of a fast food sandwich, can have a tremendous impact when it comes to losing weight. Substituting fruit instead of eating cakes will also make a difference.

Eat three meals a day and don't eat at night. You can eat raw vegetables between meals. You will find that by following this diet plan, you will not only lose weight successfully, but you will also feel better.

One thing you have to remember is to eat only until you are no longer hungry. Instead of stuffing yourself until you can no longer eat, eat until you are no longer hungry. When you feel hungry, eat something other than one of the foods you should avoid and wait 20 minutes before snacking again. Often, the signal that we are no longer hungry to travel to the brain takes some time. You don't need to starve to lose weight. You can do it and even be healthier at the same time if you follow this type of diet.

Green tea... Does it work?

There has been a lot of talk about green tea and how it can work for diets. Does green tea work to help you lose weight? Yes. As long as it's a homemade green tea, not sweetened.   If you think you can drink gallons of sweetened green tea and lose weight, think again.

Green tea has health benefits not found in black tea. In general, tea is a drink that is good for you. There are hundreds of different teas and many green teas of different flavors. You can drink green tea with caffeine or without caffeine. This acts as a diuretic and will cleanse the system. I drink green tea all day and have managed to maintain my weight after losing the weight I wanted to lose while returning to my regular diet.

While water works well as a diuretic, green tea is more stimulating. Speaking of someone who has tried both, green tea works better when it comes to losing weight than when it comes to drinking pure water. I drink decaffeinated green tea that I make myself. You end up visiting the bathroom often when you drink tea or water throughout the day, but you also manage to clean your system and maintain weight.

You should look for green tea in bags or loose that you can prepare at home. One of the most pleasant aspects of green tea is that it can be drunk hot or cold. It's easy to make iced green tea even without a tea machine. All you need is tea bags, a bowl and boiling water. Put the tea bags in the bowl, add the boiling water and let it rest for about five minutes. Then fill the rest of the container with cold water and remove the tea bags. Refresh it and you'll have iced tea that you can drink all day.

You can find green tea flavors in the grocery store that contain no calories. Natural green tea, however, is the one that works best. You should not add sugar to tea as this will defeat the purpose in drinking it.

If you don't like the taste of sugar-free green tea, then drink water. You'll find that you take the weight off the water, which is usually about five pounds, by drinking plenty of green tea or water throughout the day. Not only will it help you lose weight, but it also keeps you full. You tend to want to eat less when you drink sugar-free drinks throughout the day. In contrast, sweetened beverages, even those made with artificial sweeteners, make you want to eat more.

Stay away from canned green teas or teas sold in ready-made stores. They won't let you lose weight, but they can also help you gain weight. You can also make "tea from the sun" by putting the tea bags in cold water and putting the container in the sunlight. It is prepared naturally throughout the day and the taste is often better than if made with boiling water.

There are green diet teas that are on the market that are supposed to allow you to lose more weight. These dietary teas are usually highly concentrated in caffeine. You can get the best effects without the nerves you get by drinking too much caffeine by drinking regular green tea.

If you drink green tea with caffeine,

switch to decaffeinated green tea as the day goes by so you don't stay awake from the effects of caffeine. You may want to switch your morning drink from coffee to green tea so you can have an advantage in the day. Although both contain caffeine, coffee caffeine is more potent than green tea and less diuretic.

"Magic pills" to lose weight

There are many diet pills on the market. They make all sorts of promises, most of the time it is that you can eat whatever you want and magically lose weight by consuming these pills. Such diet pills have been sold for years and most of them, over the years, have been banned in the United States after people died or became seriously ill after taking them.

Diet pills are often nothing more than stimulants. Over-the-counter diet pills are usually caffeine tablets. They can cause a rapid heartbeat and even lead to more serious consequences for those who take them. There are fat-blocking diet pills that were very popular a few years ago. Most of them have been banned. In fact, it usually does not take a few years from the time a diet pill is introduced as the miracle cure for obesity on the market and the time it is banned because it causes liver disease or cancer.

You can lose weight without having to take any weight loss pills. I never took any diet pills because I knew people who did and had trouble taking them. Taking diet pills is similar to taking cocaine to lose weight. You're actually sacrificing your health to try to be thinner.

Why do you want to lose weight? There are two good reasons to lose weight. First and foremost, it's healthier not to be overweight. Obesity can cause many health problems, especially heart disease and diabetes. Therefore, it is naturally healthier to maintain a good weight.

The second reason is that you want to

look good. But you also want to look healthy. You want to lose weight in a healthy way that makes your body feel stronger and healthier and also increases your self-esteem. When you take off 10 pounds in 10 days, you will feel very empowered and in control of your body, even if you have more weight to use.

But you never want to compromise your health if you want to lose weight. The truth is that there is no "magic pill" that can make you lose weight. Many diet pills don't work and are just a way to take your money. Many are simply caffeine tablets that will give you a very unpleasant feeling of a racing heart (imagine drinking 6 cups of coffee at a time - that's how it feels when you take diet pills). Some of them are frankly dangerous and are still marketed online, although they are banned in the United States and other countries.

Of course, some of the slimming pills are just laxatives. Although it's important to evacuate daily to lose weight and keep it down, laxatives can overload your digestive tract. If you need laxatives, take them as directed. But never use laxatives or laxatives disguised as diet pills to lose weight.

Those who market diet pills do it to a desperate public. People who are desperate to lose weight will want to believe that they can magically lose weight without having to sacrifice anything they are currently doing.

The manufacturers of these pills will tell people anything they want to hear, including that the pills are made from herbal ingredients and that the pharmaceutical companies have a big conspiracy with the FDA to keep them out of the country. This isn't true. If the drugs are banned by the FDA, then that makes them pretty bad. Especially when considering the side effects of many of the FDA-approved drugs.

Save your money and your health and stay away from any pill that promises you results that seem too good to be true. Some ads for these pills promise that they will allow you to lose 10 pounds in 3 days. This is very unhealthy. You can easily lose 10 pounds in 10 days by following the healthy plans described in this book (which is one pound a day), but losing 10 pounds in 3 days would be a dramatic (if it worked) and unhealthy weight loss.

On top of that, you probably won't keep the weight at all. If you follow the examples in this book, you will not only lose the 10 pounds you want to lose, but you will also keep them away.

"Body Cleaners"

You've probably seen the many ads for body cleansers that are also used for weight loss. These are usually composed of water mixed with some herbs that are supposed to clean your system and allow you to lose weight. Many of these body cleaners start at $50. Save your money.

The way body cleansers, or detoxifiers as they are also called, work is to have you drink a solution and then follow it with two large glasses of water. You can get the same effect by drinking one glass of green tea and then following it with two glasses of water. You'll go to the bathroom repeatedly and empty your system.

Rinsing your system is good for weight

loss, but you don't want to exaggerate, and you certainly don't want to spend a lot of money on water. If you are interested in this form of weight loss, you can use a detox once every few days that you do it yourself. You can add herbal ingredients like lemon pepper to the water and drink it. But green tea is much nicer.

There's such a thing as drinking too much water. You don't want to overload your system with water on a regular basis, as it is bad for the kidneys. You should drink 6 to 8 glasses of green tea or water a day to lose weight or maintain weight loss. Drinking too much water can be very difficult for the kidneys.

Like diet pills, body cleansers are sold to the public as the magic way to lose weight without trying. Many of these cleaners are sold to supposedly detoxify the body against toxins and also the drugs you may be taking. You can get the same detoxification by drinking unsweetened liquids and water.

While it can be frustrating when you are trying to lose weight and you may want to come up with something that will allow you to make this easier, you are wasting your money and your time by purchasing body cleansing products to lose weight. Once again, there is no "magic" way to lose weight. Losing 10 pounds will take 10 days if you follow this healthy regimen. It will work, and what's more, you'll feel healthier. The only thing that will be heavier on you will be your pockets of money you saved from falling prey to products that are designed for those with more money than sense.

Stopping eating won't make you lose weight.

One of the ways I used to diet all the time is exceptionally unhealthy. I did this often at 40 and wondered why I couldn't lose more than 5 pounds. This is called a "starvation diet.

A friend of mine explained to me that not only is the starvation diet a dangerous form of dieting, but it is also ineffective. The starvation diet is just what it seems - not eating. Or eat a piece of bread all day. Naturally, this isn't healthy for you, but people do it anyway. The reason people use the starvation diet is because they are desperate to lose weight and feel that by not consuming calories, they will lose weight.

You can lose weight, naturally, by starving. But it'll take a long time. On top of that, you'll be unhealthy and you'll feel sick. You'll feel weak and tired all the time. You may faint. A woman in a village a few kilometres away killed a child on a bicycle because she fainted at the wheel of her car after following a starvation diet.

When I starved to death, I could lose five pounds immediately. However, this is normal in weight loss. This is the weight of the water and will come off no matter what type of diet you try. Then I got frustrated because I couldn't take off any more weight. This was because my metabolism had stopped, only I didn't know until years later.

To burn your body fat, you need to have a healthy metabolism. Your metabolism is what burns calories. For your metabolism to work properly, you need fuel. It's like a machine, with no fuel, shuts down. Just as your car doesn't run without gasoline, your metabolism doesn't run without food.

What happens when your metabolism shuts down?

When your metabolism shuts down, your body goes into "starvation mode. Your body is intelligent, much more than you think. When the body feels that it is not getting fuel, it begins to shut down, just like a machine. This means that everything starts to shut down, including your immune system.

You don't burn calories when your metabolism shuts down. You end up in a dead end when it comes to losing weight. You also discover that your immune system shuts down. That's why I always felt bad when I tried to starve to death.

Starvation diets don't work and are very unhealthy. While you may go from starvation mode and eventually start losing weight, you will be doing so at great risk to your health. Often, this kind of thinking and diet method leads to anorexia, a condition that causes someone to have a distorted view of their body and feel that if they eat something, they will become fat. This is a psychological disorder that can occur when someone feels in control, perhaps for the first time, of their weight. It will lead to a complete closure of the organs and death.

There's another reason starvation diets don't work. After a while, when your body cries out for food, you'll start to feel as if you're very weak and you'll most likely give in to temptation. You'll probably gorge yourself on something that's not good for you. Then you could try to starve yourself again. This is known as compulsive binge eating and often produces the opposite effect. You actually gained the weight you lost and something else. Besides that, you are taking risks with your health in this way.

   You can lose weight in 10 days.   You don't have to starve to do it. In fact, if you starve to death, you won't lose 10 pounds, but probably about five pounds. Then you'll feel sick and weak and most likely you'll get upset with everything and eat, gain the weight you lost and then something else.

Watch what you drink!

I used to work with a woman who complained she couldn't lose weight. She was doing all the right things - eating the right foods and exercising constantly. In fact, he seemed to eat less than I did and definitely, according to his accounts, he exercised more than I did, but he still couldn't lose weight. I figured I just had a low metabolism and mine was higher. Then, one night after work, when our group went out to dinner, I saw why it wasn't losing weight.

After her fourth cocktail, she said she was drinking more than she was used to. Apparently, he drank a few cocktails at night, every night. In fact, everyone in the department knew this woman liked to drink less of me. That's why I wasn't losing weight.

When you are on a diet to try to lose weight, you often concentrate on the foods you are eating. This is good - you need to be careful what you eat when you're trying to lose weight. But you also have to be careful what you drink.

Every time I wanted to lose five pounds in a week without really getting to work, I skipped the cream and sugar in my coffee. This simple thing allowed me to lose weight. I didn't put so much sugar in my coffee or my cream. But I realized that sugar is really an enemy of those who are trying to lose weight.

The alcohol is full of sugar. People think they can drink wine and get away with it by drinking and still lose weight. While red wine may be good for you in some capacity, it is not good for you when you are trying to lose weight. No alcohol is good for you - everything contains sugar. Some of them contain more sugar than others. Mixed drinks, such as cocktails, usually contain more sugar. Beer has a high sugar content. White wine has a high sugar content. The lowest sugar content that can be obtained in alcohol comes from a very dry red wine. But you should still avoid it when you're trying to lose weight.

Soda's off limits. It's nothing but liquid candy. Even diet sodas are bad for you and don't promote weight loss, but weight gain. Carbonation in the soda leads to weight addition and hinders weight loss efforts. You should not drink diet sodas or soda when you are trying to lose weight.

Milk is high in fat and must be off limits. Juices, although some of them are good for you, are high in sugar and off limits when you are on a weight loss diet. You should look at the juices anyway, as many of them contain very little fruit juice and a lot of sugar.

Energy drinks and sports drinks are also high in sugar and should be avoided when it comes to losing weight. You should drink nothing but water and maybe coffee and black tea when you are looking for a way to lose weight.

It's just as important to watch what you drink as what you eat when you're on a diet. You may be consuming hundreds of calories a day with what you drink. The reason my colleague at work couldn't lose weight was because he consumed more than the caloric content his body needed through his alcohol consumption. I was never going to lose weight while I was still drinking.

For some people, a simple change to water from their daily drinks can make all the difference in the world when it comes to losing weight. I met a woman who drank a lot of cola who switched to water and claimed she had lost 30 pounds in a month just for making this simple lifestyle change.

If you want to lose weight, you should not only watch what you eat, but also what you drink. Water, sugar-free coffee and sugar-free tea have no calories. Drink this only and stay away from so-called diet drinks, as these will prohibit your efforts to lose weight.

I'm so sorry... But you really need to get some exercise.

Dieting without exercise is a complete waste of time. Remember when we talked about metabolism? It accelerates when you exercise. Exercise will not only help you burn fat and promote weight loss, but it will also make you feel more energetic and emotionally healthy. If you think you can lose weight, think again. You need exercise to lose weight.

The type of exercise you do is also important. You need to do cardiovascular exercises to lose weight. Cardio exercise makes your heart pump and your metabolism work. These are exercises like the following:

- Run
- Walking speed
- Jogging
- Elliptical training
- Staircase with steps
- Rowing
- Jump
- Dancing

All of this causes your heart rate to increase and helps you burn calories. While toning and yoga exercises are a good way to relax, cardiovascular exercises are a good way to get energy and burn fat. This is why you need to make them as early in the day as possible.

You should set the alarm 15 minutes early and exercise in the morning. You don't have to buy expensive gym equipment for your home. You don't have to buy a gym membership, though this isn't a bad idea. All you have to do is start your heart in the morning by exercising and raising your metabolism. When you combine cardiovascular exercise with protein in the morning, you're preparing your metabolism to burn calories during the day. By simply adding 15 minutes of exercise in the morning, you can easily take off 10 pounds in 10 days.

When you start exercising for the first time, you can start slowly. Never try too hard or get to a point where you feel bad. If you get dizzy while exercising or feel pain, stop. You can start by walking at a brisk pace or even jogging lightly into place in the morning. Any little exercise you can do and don't normally do will help you lose weight by increasing your metabolism.

Don't think you'll get tired of exercising. Just the opposite. You'll have more energy when you exercise than when you don't. That's why you shouldn't do cardiovascular exercise at night before going to bed.

If you can't do cardiovascular exercise when you wake up in the morning, you should do it when you get home at night. You should wait at least 20 minutes after eating to exercise and never just before going to bed. If you are looking for a way to relax at night and also tone your muscles, giving you a better shape, you can do Pilates. These are stretching exercises that can help your body get in shape while relaxing you at the same time. Yoga exercises are also good for exercising before going to bed.

Running in place is a good way to get your heart pumping in the morning and doesn't require you to buy any equipment or spend money on a gym. You can run in your place as soon as you get out of bed in the morning and then jump up and down to get your heart going. The more exercise you do, the easier it will be. You'll find that every day, it gets a little easier and you have more energy. Once you get into an exercise routine, it's like an addiction. The more exercise you do, the easier it will be and the more fit you will feel. As you begin to see results, you'll want to exercise even more.

Exercise not only helps you lose weight, but also promotes body toning. As you lose fat, you need to do something about your skin. You don't want it to fall, so by exercising, you can tone your muscles and tighten your skin.

You'll also feel healthier mentally when you exercise. Many people who need to lose weight become depressed. Some people are actually depressed, which is why they are overweight: they eat from a source of comfort. Exercise actually increases the serotonin in the brain and makes you feel better. Taking a brisk walk will help you feel happier. This is compared to the effects of an antidepressant.

Don't try to lose weight without exercising. You don't have to do much, just 15 minutes a day will be enough to make an impact on your weight loss. If you combine the above recommendations for food and drink with 15 minutes of exercise in one day, you can easily lose 10 pounds in 10 days.

The important thing is not only what you eat, but also how you eat it.

It's not only what you eat that can cause you to gain weight or not lose it, but also the way you eat. My father, for example, complained that he couldn't lose weight, even though he never ate breakfast or lunch and only ate dinner. The reason she couldn't lose weight was because she consumed all her calories at once, at the end of the day, and didn't give her metabolism time to act when it came to burning calories. His metabolism was off all day and only came to life at night. When it soon went out again when he went to sleep.

You need to eat three meals a day to lose weight, breakfast being the most important. It's better to eat most calories at breakfast than at any other time. This will allow your body to use the fuel you give it to burn calories during the day. If you consume calories at night, you are not allowing your body to burn them. When my father started eating three times a day, he started losing weight.

In addition to eating three meals a day, you should stop eating before bedtime. When you eat before going to bed, not only can it cause indigestion, but it stays in your system and does not burn. You shouldn't eat anything before going to bed. Give yourself a time limit and look for something other than to eat before going to bed. You may want to make a lifestyle change by doing yoga or stretching while watching TV so you're not tempted to eat snacks. Many people sit in front of the TV and eat snacks before going to bed, which contributes greatly to obesity in our society.

Also watch your portions. For example, you should never eat directly from the potato chip bag. Although you may want to avoid potato chips when dieting, after dieting and losing weight, you may want to eat potato chips. This isn't a big crime, but you should be careful with your portions. If you pour the chips into a small bowl, you can control your portions.

Remember the fact that it often takes the brain time to register when we are full. Many people eat out of habit and think they are hungry, when in fact they are not. You should always wait 20 minutes after eating before eating again. This gives the brain time to record the fact that you are full.

Simply cutting the portions in half can also help you lose weight. Too often, we eat until we feel like we're about to explode. This isn't good. The secret to maintaining a healthy weight is to eat until you're no longer hungry, not until you're satisfied. You should never strive to have that uncomfortable feeling of fullness.

You should also eat at the same time every day. If you keep a good meal schedule, you'll have a better digestive system. People who eat regularly and at a certain time tend to see that their digestive system works the same way every day. This eliminates constipation which can also cause swelling and weight gain. You should have a bowel movement once a day and usually at the same time every day. This leads to good weight control and helps you lose weight. It also keeps your digestive tract healthy.

Chew your food well. Many people have

a habit of eating their food. You should not only do this to promote weight loss, but also to help your digestive system. Large pieces of food are harder to digest than smaller particles. He also tends to eat more when he doesn't chew his food well. Chewing your food 20 times is an old diet trick that still works. You will find that this gives your stomach time to signal to your mind when it is full and you do not overeat.

Drink a glass of water before each meal. This also makes you feel full and allows you to eat less. By drinking a glass of water before each meal and chewing your food well, you will find that you are eating less and losing weight. If you only have 10 pounds to lose, these two tips alone can go a long way toward helping you lose weight.

Losing weight doesn't have to mean a

drastic lifestyle or a new diet. Usually, you can lose weight by just taking a look at your eating habits and making some changes. Be sure to watch how you eat as much as what you eat and you'll find those 10 pounds come off easily.

The importance of your age

As you age, your metabolism begins to decline. This is why older people often complain that they have more difficulty trying to lose weight than younger people.

Older people have to accept the fact that they are not going to have the body they had when they were 20. They'll probably be a little milder when it comes to their weight. But that doesn't give them carte blanche to explode like a balloon.

To know your ideal weight, you need to know your age, as well as your height and bone structure. You can look at any chart in the doctor's office to see that your age correlates with your ideal weight, as does your sex.

As you age, because your metabolism is slowing down, you'll need less food. One mistake people make as they age is that they continue to consume the same amount of calories as when they were younger. You need more exercise and less food when you grow up to stay fit.

If you have children, it may be harder to maintain weight as you grow when you give birth. It's much harder for a 35-year-old woman to lose weight than it is for a 25-year-old woman. You have to work very hard because the metabolism tends to decrease as we age.

The methods used in this book to lose 10 pounds in 10 days are made for someone over 40 years old. Those who are younger and have a higher metabolism can lose more than 10 pounds in 10 days by following the advice in this book. If you're reading this and you think you can't lose weight because it's bigger, think again. If I can do it, so can you. I know a lot of people who have tried this kind of lifestyle change (I don't like to call it a diet) and have lost weight. Whether you have 10 pounds to lose or need to lose a lot more weight, this diet will work well for you, regardless of your age.

Discover your ideal weight

Do you know what your ideal weight is? You can find out how much you should weigh for your height, age, and sex based on a chart. There are online charts that you can use to determine your ideal weight.

It is important that anyone who is trying to lose weight determine their ideal weight because people often have a distorted view of what they should weigh. If your clothes are tight and you want to lose 10 pounds, then you can easily do it in 10 days using the tips in this book. If you are overweight and need to know how much you need to lose to reach your ideal weight, then you can calculate how much weight you need to lose to reach your goal.

Don't be discouraged if you need to lose more than 10 pounds. If you follow the instructions in this book, you can lose as much weight as you want safely and quickly. However, you should set goals when it comes to losing weight.

Instead of focusing on the final goal, you should have a goal each week when it comes to how much weight you can lose. You can lose 5 pounds a week if you work on this program. This is a safe amount of weight to lose.

If you join programs like Jenny Craig or Weight Watchers, you should keep in mind that their goal is to make money. Both organizations offer counseling and Jenny Craig provides the food you eat. But both are business. They'll tell you you have to lose 2 pounds a week. This keeps you coming back to them longer than you need.

The information found in this book combines the basic concept of Weight Watchers (a very good diet plan that makes sense) with diet recommendations, as well as tips for eating and exercising. The goal of this book is to help you lose 10 pounds in 10 days, but you can continue to follow the tips for losing more weight if you need to.

If you set a goal aside each week and weigh yourself once a week, you will reach your final goal. One of the biggest mistakes a dieter makes is to become discouraged and abandon the concept of weight loss. This often happens when someone reaches a plateau and cannot lose any more weight. What you need to do then is change your diet and try something new to lose weight. Don't be discouraged, as you can lose the weight you want and keep it off by simply following the instructions in this book.

Understanding your ideal weight will help you feel more confident in your weight loss goals. If you have a lot of weight to lose, this book will help you start your diet and also give you the instructions you need to take off the rest of your weight. You shouldn't be discouraged if you cheat on your diet or gain a pound. Just push it back into the past, where it belongs, and move on when you try to reach your ideal weight.

Conclusion: The power of mind over matter

The biggest secret to losing weight lies in your own mind. Losing weight is like quitting smoking - no one can make you do it - you have to want to do it for yourself. If you want to quit smoking, you can quit the package and walk away from it without looking back. I know... I did this. The same goes for weight loss.

Your mind is more powerful than anything else. If you want to lose weight, you can do it yourself. Weight loss cannot be due to a suggestion from a doctor or someone else - it's all up to you. One of the reasons why organizations like Weight Watchers are so popular is that they force someone to take responsibility for their weight. By going to meetings and being heavy, you feel compelled to lose weight. You can give yourself the same sense of obligation and save money and time by putting your mind above matter.

In short, your desire to want to lose weight has to exceed your desire to eat foods and drink beverages that are bad for you. You have to want to lose more weight than you want to eat. If you have this mentality, you can accomplish anything.

One way to motivate yourself is to look at your clothes. My motivation was to wear my thin jeans and thin shorts. This was the carrot that hung in front of me to keep me on track and lose the weight I had lost.

Every time I thought about eating something that was bad for me, like a chocolate bar, for example, I had to think about those shorts. The desire to lose weight outweighed the desire to eat candy. It was hard for me (and probably for most people) because I live in a house with two skinny kids who like Oreo cookies and other things I also like to eat. I couldn't put them on a diet too by getting rid of everything that was tempting in the house, so I had to do it alone.

However, if you live with others who are overweight, you may consider helping the whole family catch up when it comes to eating the right foods. Eliminating some of the foods your family eats will not only help you with your weight loss goals, but also with them. This can be a healthy ideal for the whole family.

If you live alone, it's easier to give up some of the treats that may tempt you with your diet. You can simply choose not to buy them. When they're not in the house, you're not tempted to eat them. Or drink them.

You should keep your motivation positive rather than negative. Instead of thinking about how you don't fit into your clothes, think about how good you'll look when you fit into your clothes. This positive attitude will help you stay on track and work wonders when it comes to losing weight.

By following the tips in this book, you can lose weight. You don't have to buy any special food. You don't have to sign up for a gym. You don't have to buy expensive drinks or take diet pills. You just need to understand how your body works, what you should eat and what you shouldn't eat and do some exercise. This is simple advice, but it works perfectly when it comes to losing weight. Above all, you need to stay positive, not give up if you think of eating a cookie, and maintain the desire to be your ideal weight over the desire to eat.

Now yes, I wish you the best in your results, and remember, everything is practical; theory without action is of no use to you. It brings everything you learn into real life.

A big hug, your friend, Jessy!